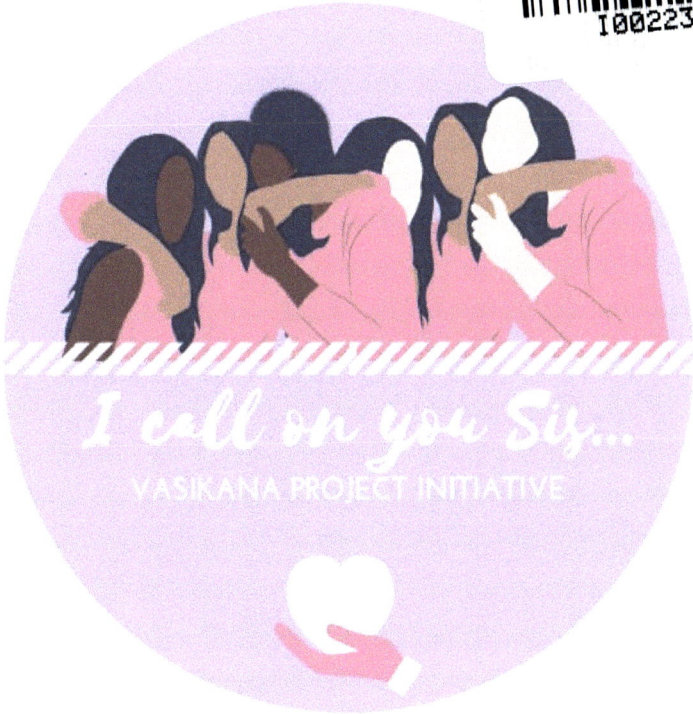

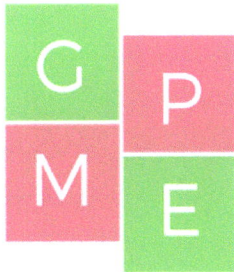

I call on you Sis...

VASIKANA PROJECT INITIATIVE

G P M E

Vasikana PROJECT

GIRLS. PUBERTY. MENSTRUATION. EMPOWERMENT

Interior design & layout by Clara Matonhodze Strode
Cover design by Clara Matonhodze Strode
Illustrated by Clara Matonhodze Strode using canva.com

Interior photos from Pexels.com
Author photograph by Karen Marie Jenkins

Printed in the United States of America
Second Printing, 2020
ISBN 978-1-970063-15-8
Library of Congress Control Number 2019910518

Ordering Information: Special discounts are available on quantity purchases by
bookstores, corporations, associations, and others. For details, contact the
publisher at sales@braughlerbooks.com or at 937-58-BOOKS.

For questions or comments about this book, please write to
multiculturalsolutionsllc@gmail.com

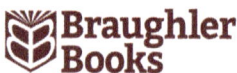

Braughler Books

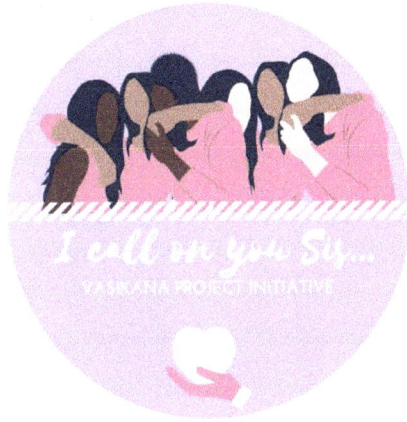

Dedication

To my sisters, who came from the same womb as me.
My sisters from another mother whose circles I stand, uplifting
me. My older sisters, grandmothers, aunts on whose shoulders I
stand; who have poured wisdom into me. My little Sisters,
daughters, and nieces following behind, who inspire me to be a
better person every day.

My heartbeats – Honest, Panashe, Hama, Nama, whose support
is unwavering.

I love you dearly.

– Zvisinei Dzepasi Mamutse –

CONTENTS

• • •

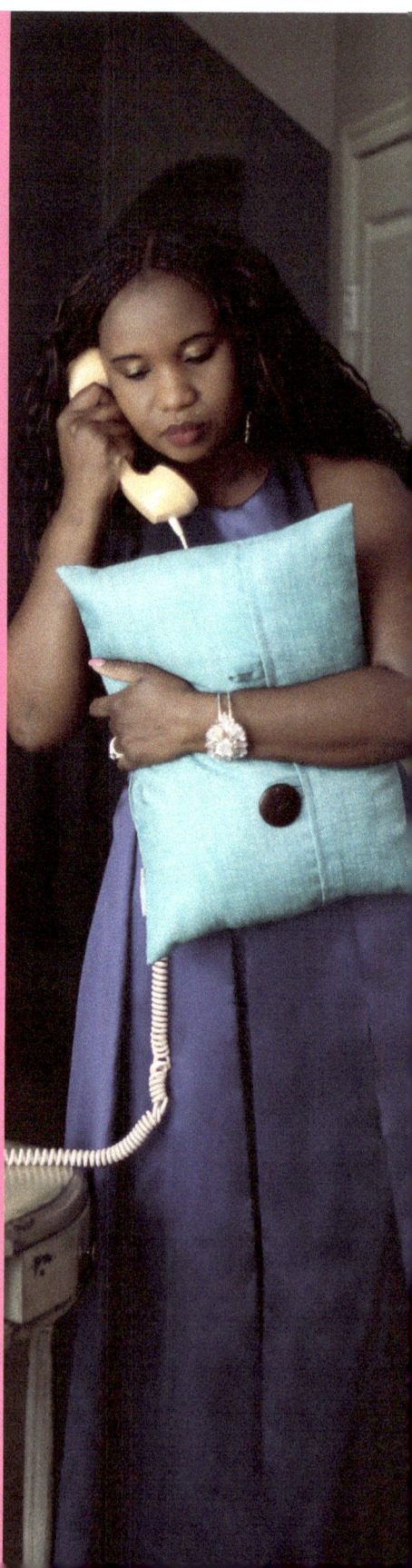

From the Author's Heart

Woman to woman, sister to sister, we call on each other to share our triumphs, struggles, dreams for ourselves, our spouses, or our children, our aspirations, encouragement, our hopes and fears. Most of all prayers for each other. Together there is nothing we cannot go through.

We rely on the older women, on whose shoulders we stand drawing wisdom from them. On the circle of women in whose circle we stand, fingers intertwined sharing strength. On the young women coming behind us, looking up to us.

I Call on You Sis, is a reminder of how these relationships are so important, in days of uncertainty, depression, and suicide; I hope Sis, you find the courage to reach out and when you are called upon, I hope too Sis, that you fan flames and not blow them out. That you build and not tear down, a life could be hanging to your every word.

Let's hold each other's fragile hearts safely in the palms of our hands.

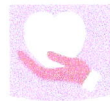

– Zvisinei Dzepasi Mamutse –

How to Use This Journal

This Journal is meant to be fun, inspiring, and a call to all women and girls to reach out to each other as they do life. Often as women, we think the challenges we face are unique to ourselves. We don't celebrate our successes enough because we don't want to brag. We live our lives in quiet desperation.

This Journal encourages you to reach out to others instead of going through life alone. You don't have to start at the beginning, scroll through and see where your emotions land you for that day. Some statements will resonate with you more than others. For those that do not, simply move on to a statement you connect with at that moment. Let's hold each other's fragile hearts safely in the palms of our hands.

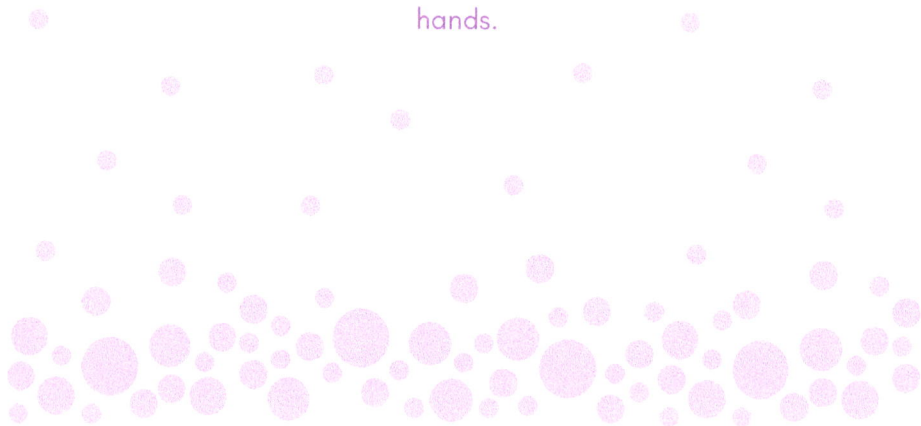

If You're the Sister Called...

Your response to a call from a fellow Sister is essential to building and empowering that Sister.

Your support and nurture are needed, and maybe for the long haul.

Before you make any promises to be there for a Sister, make sure you are emotionally available for them.

Suggest another Sister who might be able to answer a Sister's call if you cannot.

Whatever you do, do not make any commitments you are unable to keep.

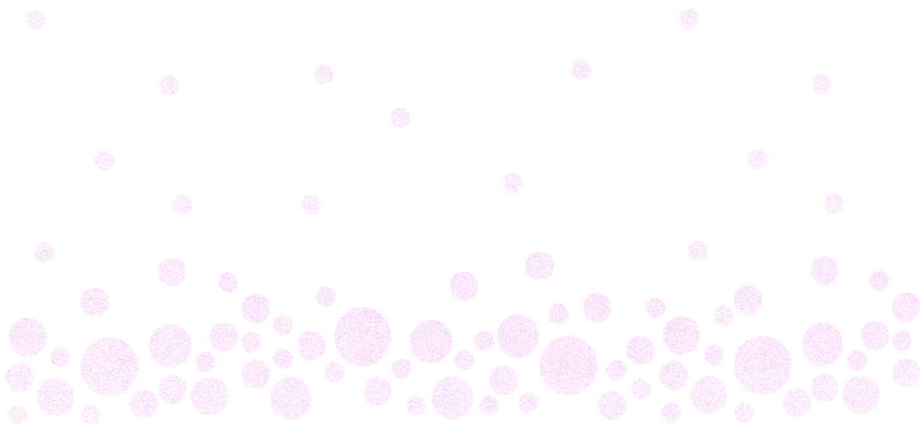

– Foreword –

Sisterhood is a special place of safety and love!

I am so pleased that Zvisinei has taken her message and lifestyle of sisterhood-love and the Dreamwalking® process from her heart, to her head, to her hands and now to her feet, to walk in her purpose, creating the "I Call On You Sis" Journal.

This special journal will not only remind generations of girls and women how important our relationships are, but also will empower school girls in Zimbabwe through puberty education.
We were all created to love and be loved and sisterhood allows us to fulfill our life's destiny!

Sonia Jackson Myles
Founder & CEO, The Sister Accord® LLC
Founder & Doula Of Dreams,
Dreamwalking®Leadership & Entrepreneurship Program

Before You Start

To find this journal useful, be with the mindset that you will be mindful of Sisterhood from now on.

♥

Before you call on a Sister, be clear about what you need help with. Focus only on your challenge and not on the challenges of others.

♥

Do not call on a Sister to spread gossip. It can be tough to not talk about the juicy details. Refocus that to finding a silver lining or to seek understanding.

♥

If you are the Sister called upon, do not hijack the conversation by talking about your own story. Be an active listener.

♥

Always remember to be mindful in all conversations. Awareness is imperative to creating a healthy Sisterhood. Honesty never goes out of style.

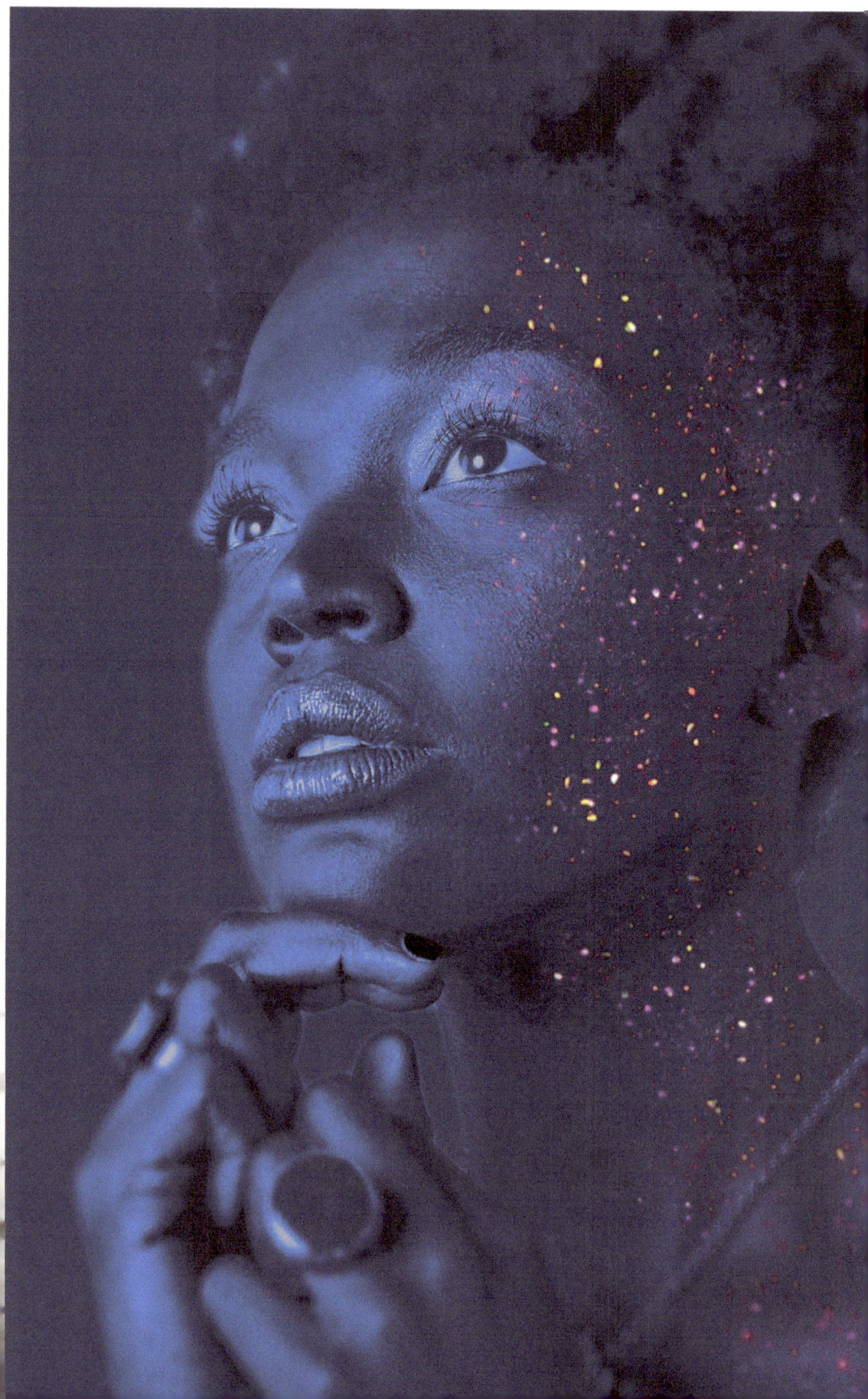

I call on You Sis...

... in my loss, and the pain becomes too hard to bear, and tears no longer fall. You, my Sis, help me realize that those we love do not go away, but continue to walk beside us, unseen.

Write about things left unsaid to a loved one who passed away. If you could see them today, what would you like them to know?

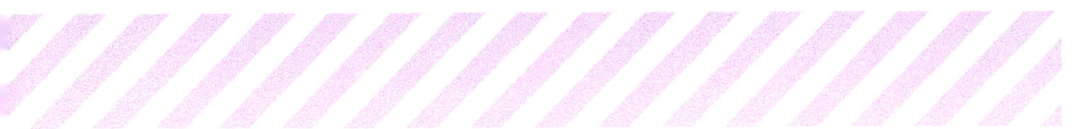

DATE:

_Grief can take care of itself, but to get
the full value of a joy you must have
somebody to divide it with._ - Mark Twain

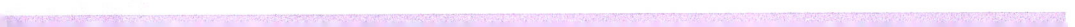

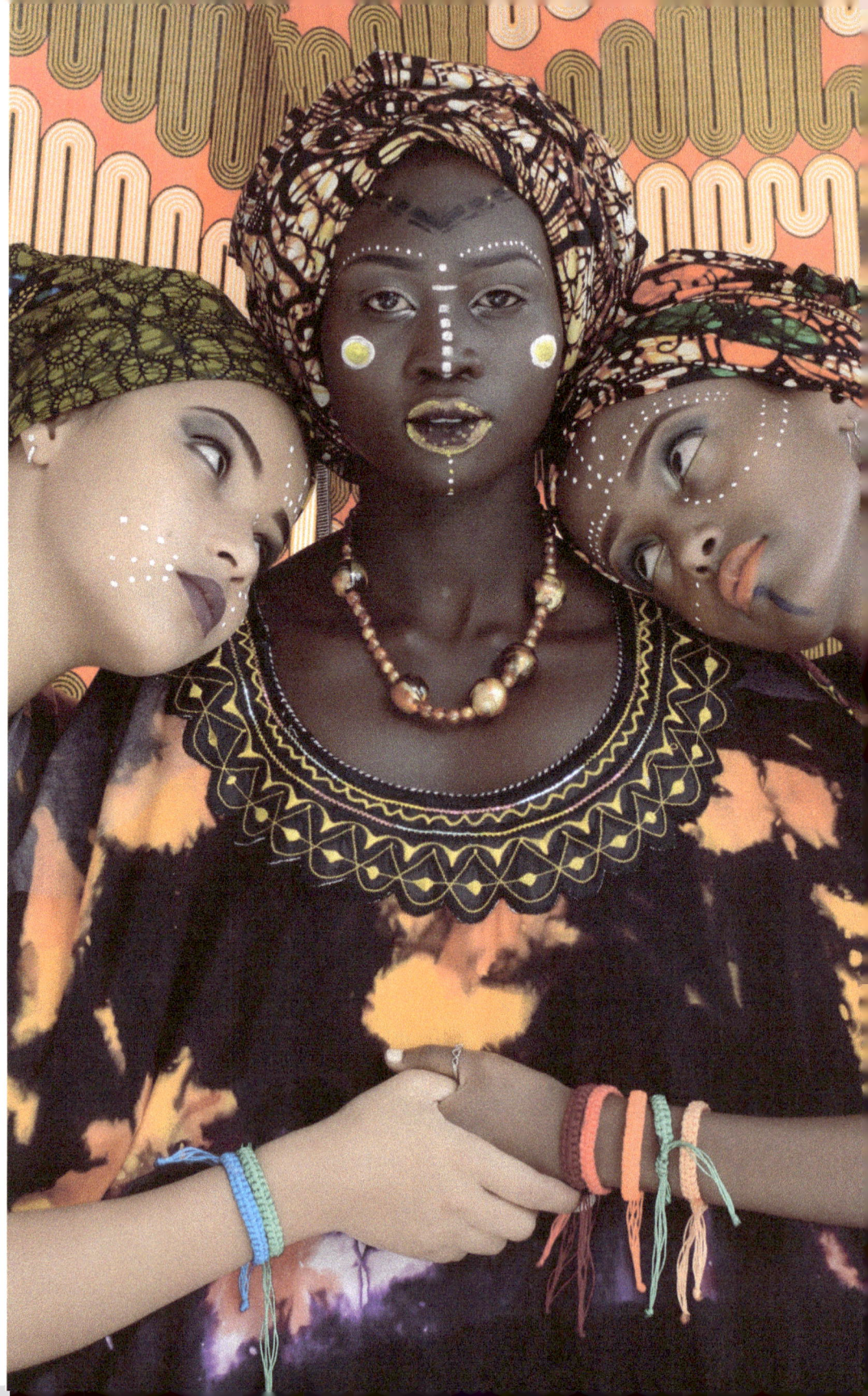

I call on You Sis...

...when I'm feeling alone because the walls in my home are closing in on me. Simply be there, not to fix anything, just to be reminded that I am not alone.

There is comfort knowing you do not have to face challenges alone. If you could speak to someone right now, write what you would say to them.
Jotting down your thoughts might help to clarify the feelings you have.

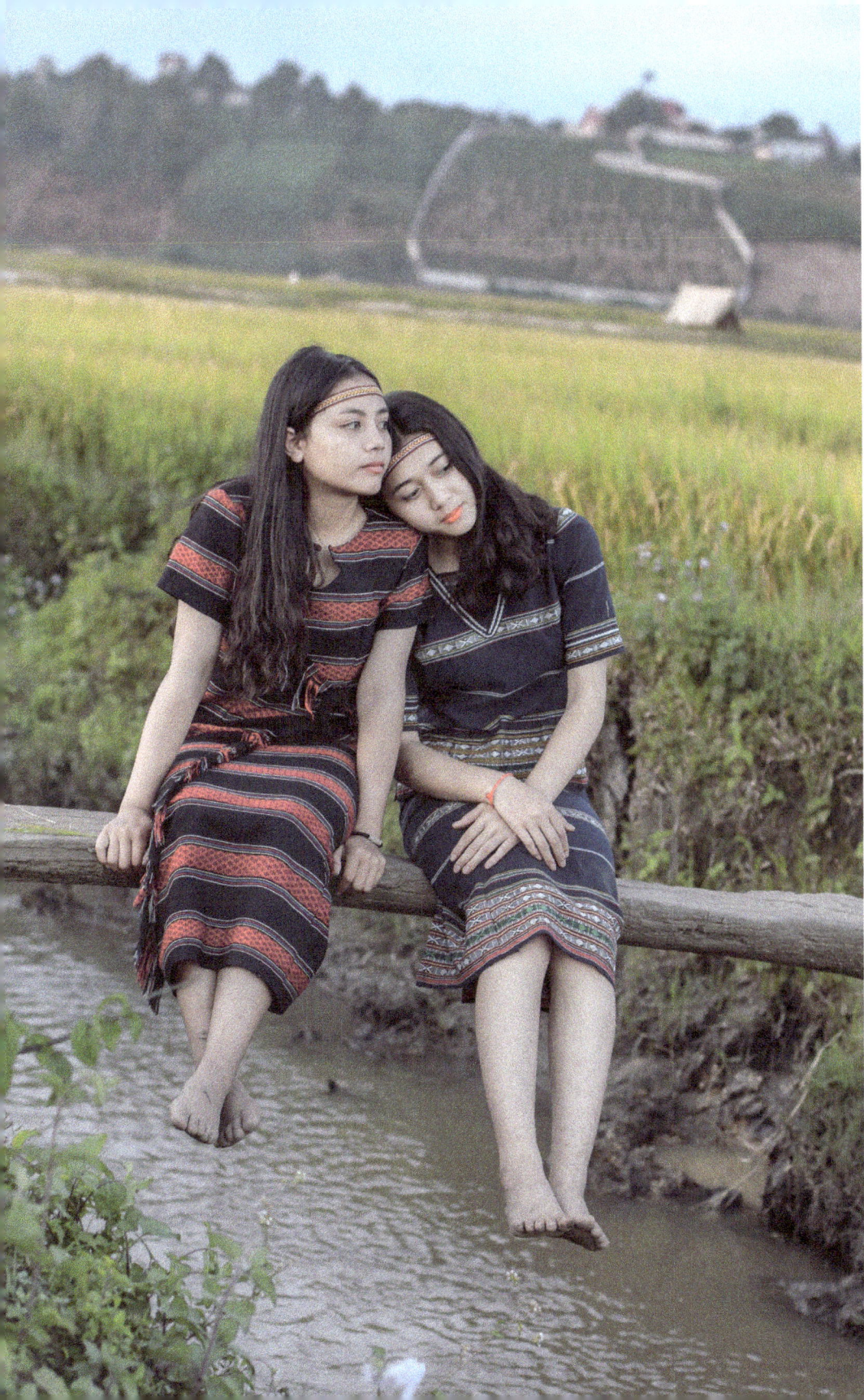

I call on You Sis...

...you are all the therapy that I need.

If you could have any type of therapy, what would it be?

Write about it and how you visualize a successful outcome from the therapy.

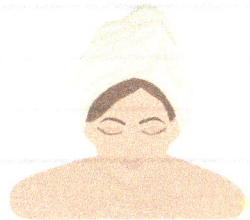

Two things I do for maintenance: I get a manicure once a month, and I see my therapist about every six weeks. I am happy to report that, at this point, my nails crack more often than I do.
- Gina Barreca

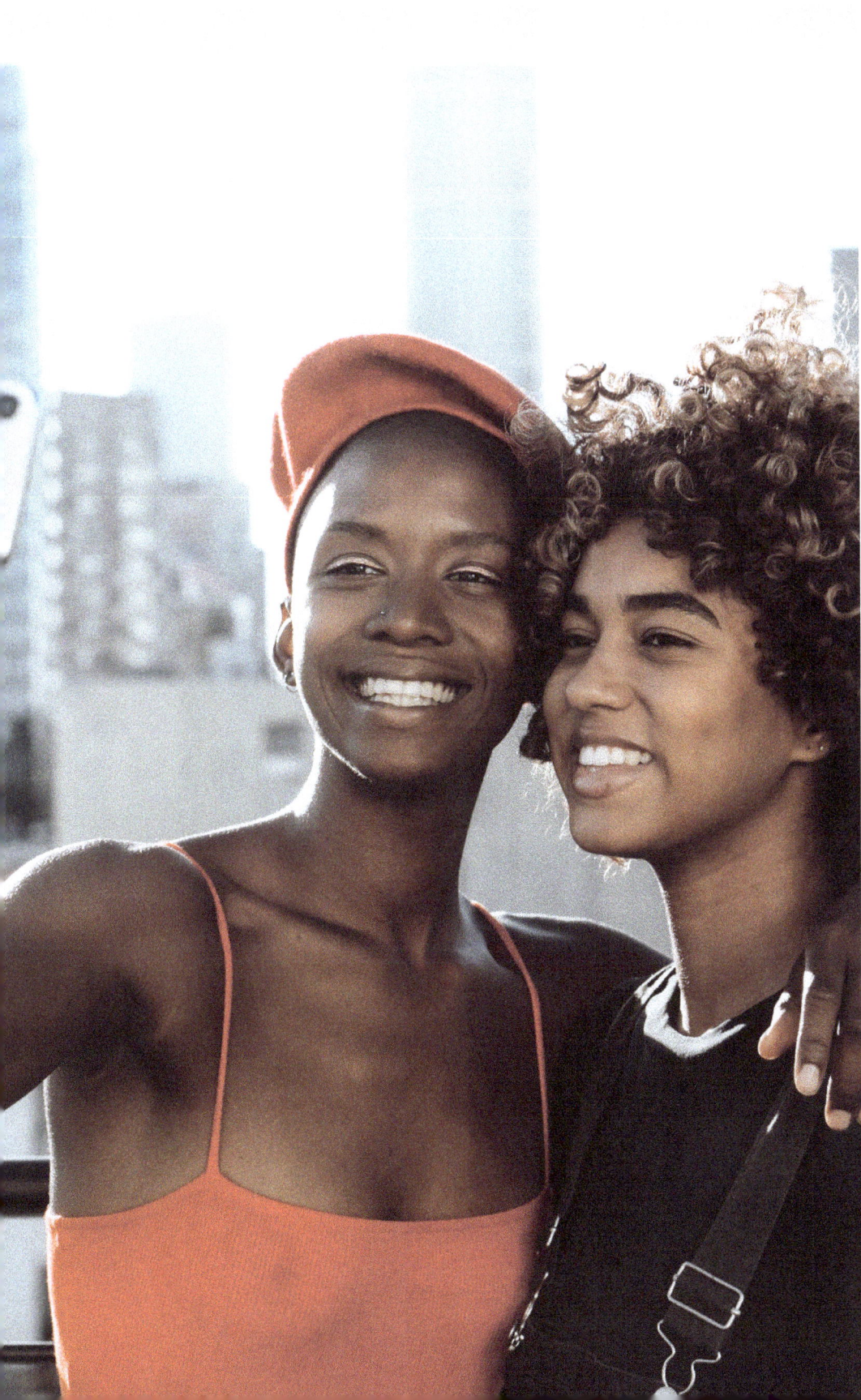

I call on You Sis...

...when my mind is foggy, and I can't make sense of it all, somehow your voice gives me clarity.

Our minds are complex.
Sometimes we hold ourselves prisoners, unable to break from toxic inner monologues. A change in perspective might hold the key to your freedom. Think about the wildest possible, but positive outcome to this situation. Write it down. How can you make it possible for you?

The only thing you sometimes have control over is perspective. You don't have control over your situation. But you have a choice about how you view it.
Chris Pine

I call on You Sis...

...when I feel weary, tired and worn out.
I tap strength from your voice.

Have you noticed how energy feeds from one person to the next? Positivity can be infectious. Write about a person you know who always has positive spirits. What do you admire about them? How do you feel when you are around them? How can you tap into their energy?

You're going to go through tough times - that's life. But I say, 'Nothing happens
to you, it happens for you.' See the positive in negative events.
Joel Osteen

I call on You Sis...

...when I have passed the point of reasoning, and I have reached the boiling point. Your calmness helps me to simmer down.

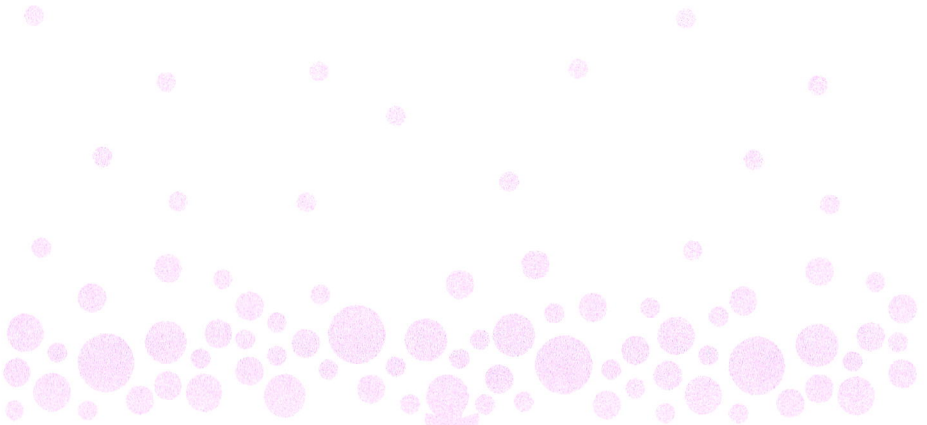

Be mindful of which flame to fan. Think of a time someone called you angry and mad. How did you react? Write about the feeling you are having now. Explore the roots of the anger and write about them.

DATE:

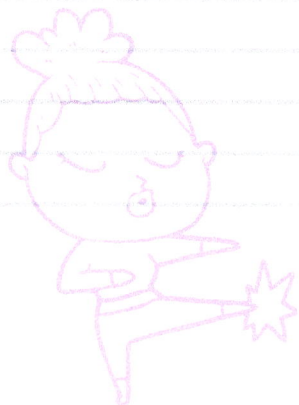

I call on You Sis...

...when a sense of loss grips me.
Leaving me torn into pieces. In you
I find comfort, and you help me
cope.

Finding the right comforting words can be difficult. We are often at a loss of how to reassure our loved ones that we are there. Write about what comforts you. Think of music, books, cafes that create your ideal escape. Describe them in great detail.

I call on You Sis...

...when I am afraid and the world seems scary, in our talks I find refuge.

So much rage is around us. Depression, suicide, and general hopelessness. How can you be a haven to others? Write about the many ways you can be a change agent that provides refuge to others.

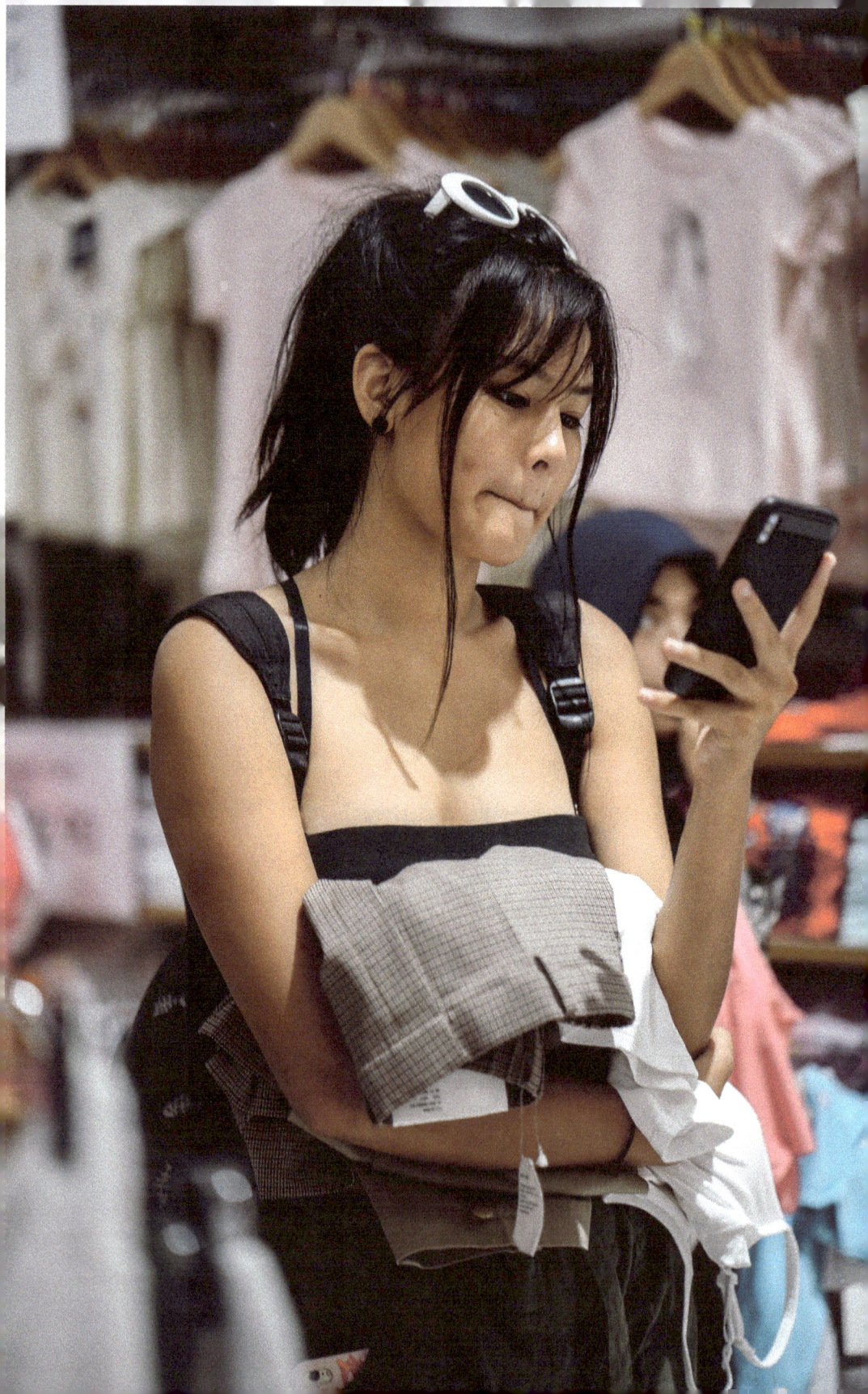

I call on You Sis...

...when my debt mounts, and
the finances dwindle. You
always help me figure out a
solution.

It takes courage for someone to call for help. It's even harder when finances are involved. Write about good spending habits that you commit to starting. What might have stopped the crisis you now face? Could it have been avoided?

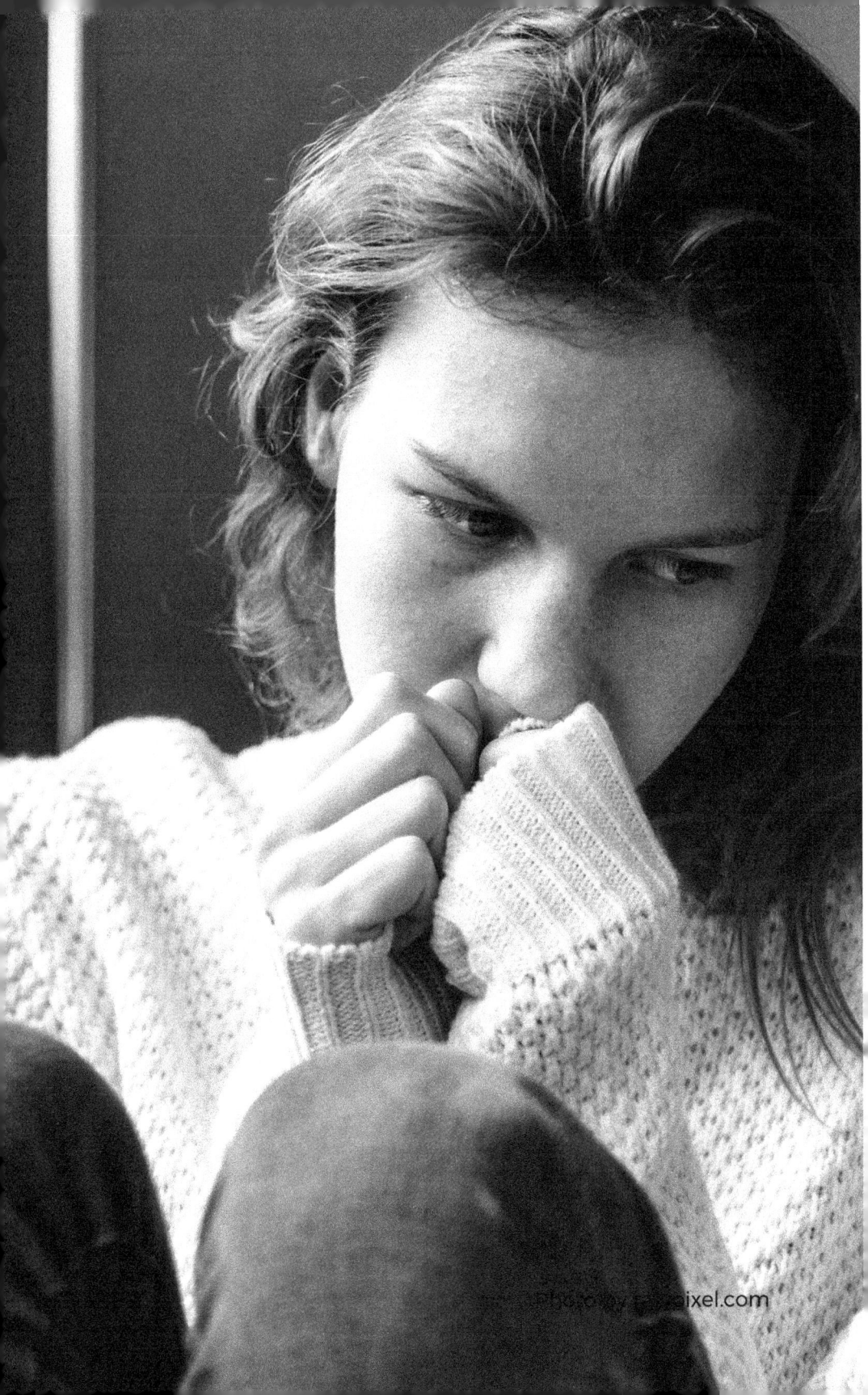

I call on You Sis...

...when I first notice the blood, and I
know deep down in my heart that my
baby is no more.
You help me process it all.

A miscarriage is one of the most painful losses a woman can go through. Sit in the pain for a while. Allow yourself to grieve and feel the loss. Write about your thoughts and feelings, and find comfort in the company of those you value.

DATE:

I call on You Sis...

...in times of loss, when my heart aches for
what was meant to be.
You wipe my tears and give me comfort.

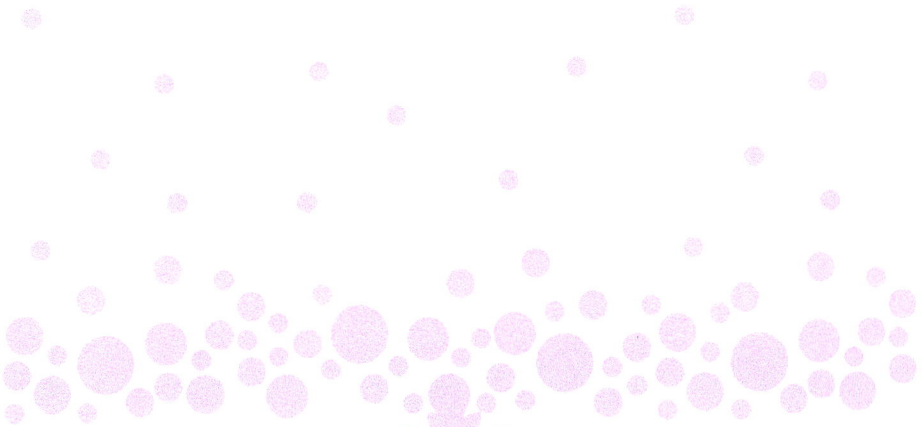

Divorce, separation and breakups are never easy for us and those in our circle. Be mindful of the pain all around. Write about the silver lining in this cloud. What does it look like?

_I used to think that divorce meant failure,
but now I see it more as a step along the
path of self-realization and growth._
Alana Stewart

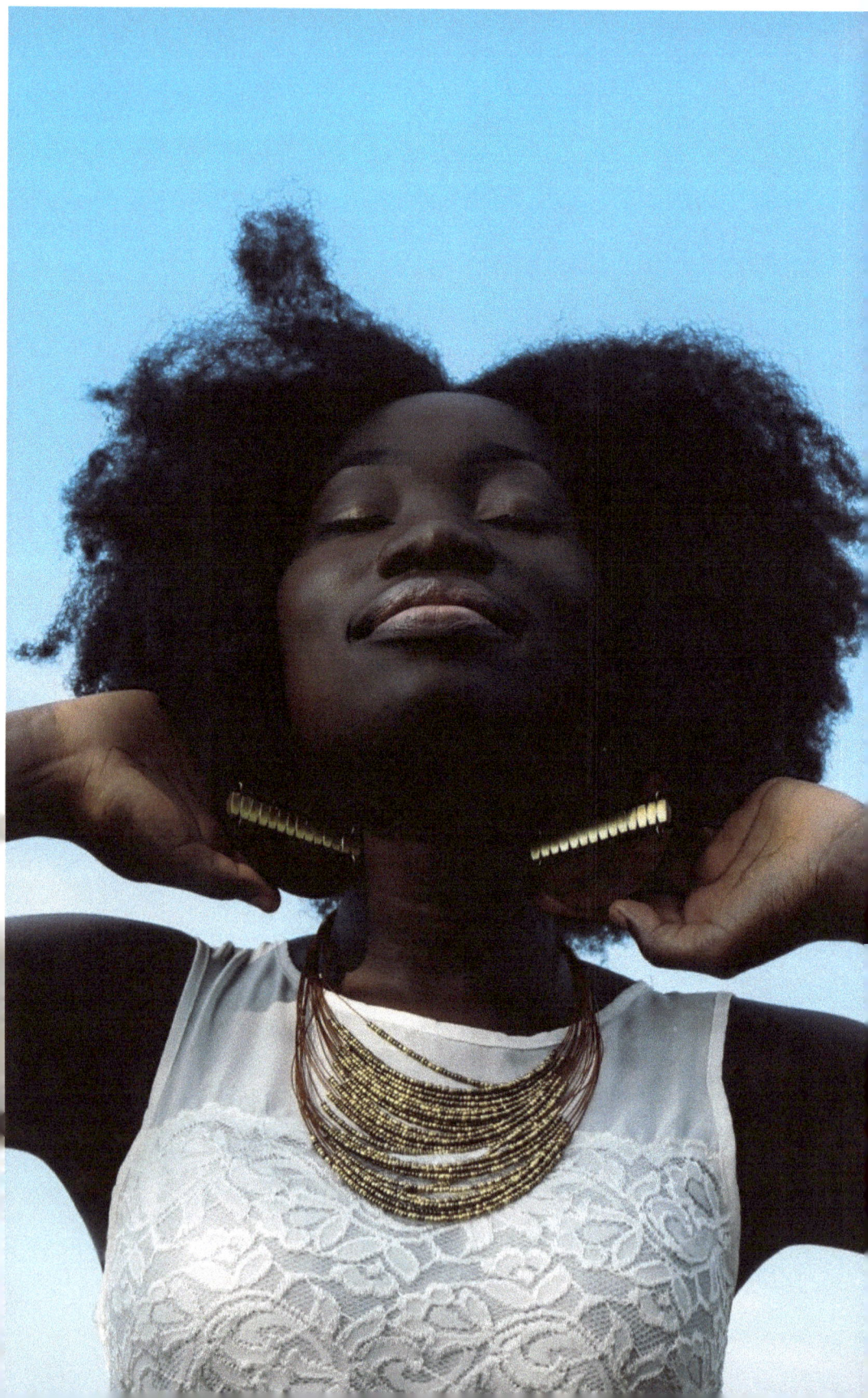

I call on You Sis...

...when storms are raging, winds blowing, rains
pouring down;
you bring me peace and calm.

In those times when life seems to be on a war path with you, take time to sit in a quiet place and evaluate your decisions. Write about your decision making process. Is it informed? how can it be better?

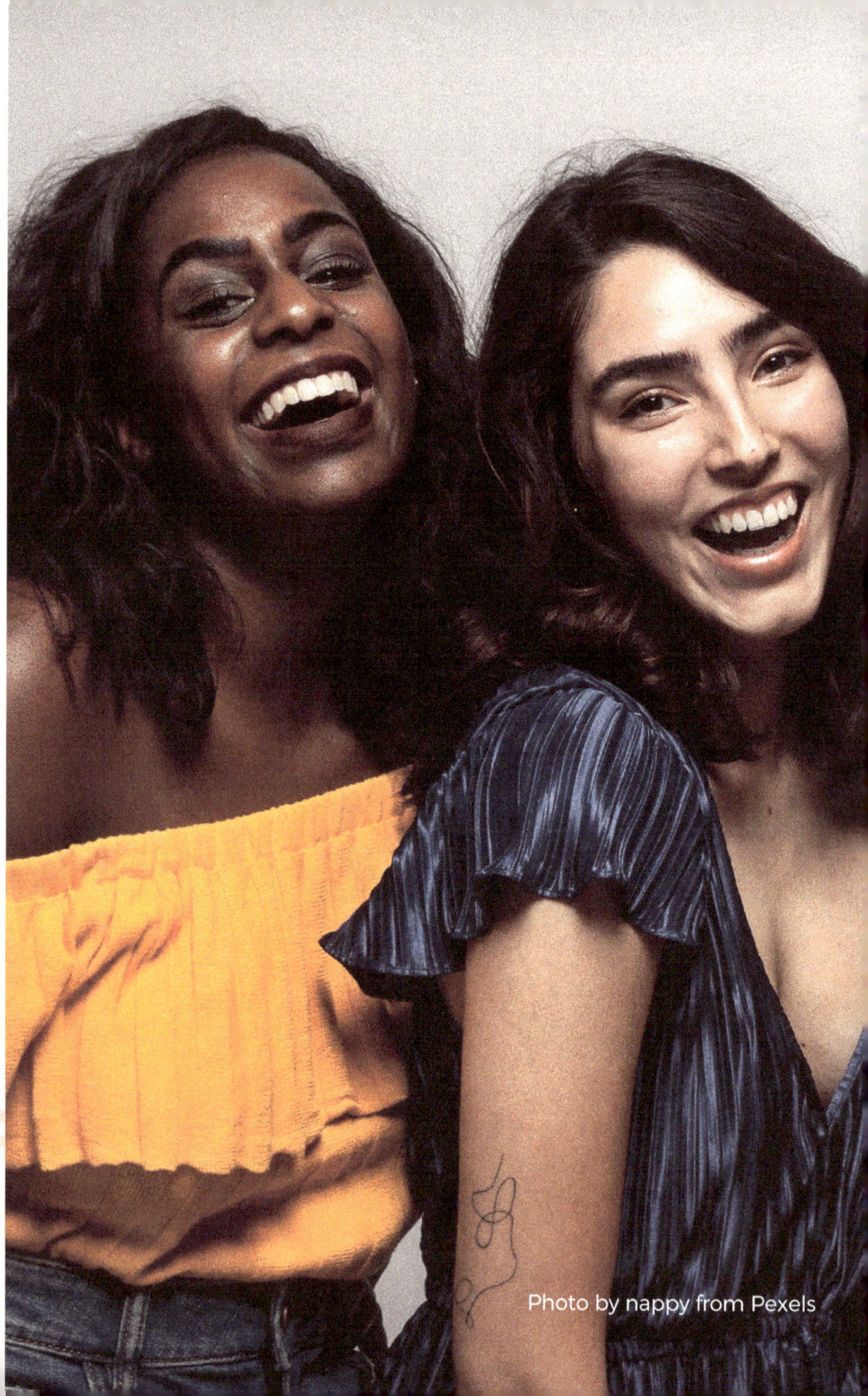

I call on You Sis...

...when I am down, you just know how to get this girl to throw her head back, laugh till I ache, you are that girl.

Laughter is the best medicine of all. Write about what made you laugh so hard. Bookmark this page, and reach for it the next time you need a good laugh.

I call on You Sis...

...when my work seems hard and dry,
you give me the energy to keep
trudging along.

There is no greater feeling than knowing you are not alone. We are in this life together and sometimes we just have to do what needs to be done. Write about what your perfect occupation looks like? what would it take to go after it? what's keeping you from pursuing your dream career?

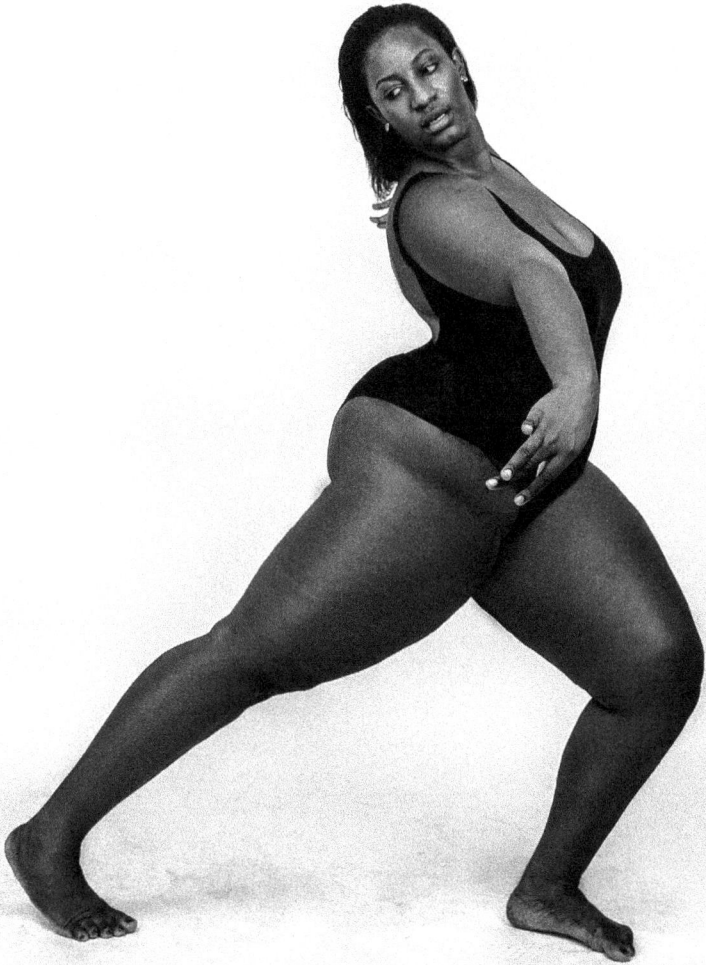

I call on You Sis...

...when my body fails me and
leaves me with scars, you help me
accept the new me.

Illness or injury can leave us scarred, imperfect and uncomfortable. However, remember inner beauty is more important. Take time to make a soul collage by creating images of aspirations, talents and dreams.

My relationship with my body has changed. I used to consider it as a servant who should obey, function, give pleasure. In sickness, you realise that you are not the boss. It is the other way around.
Federico Fellini

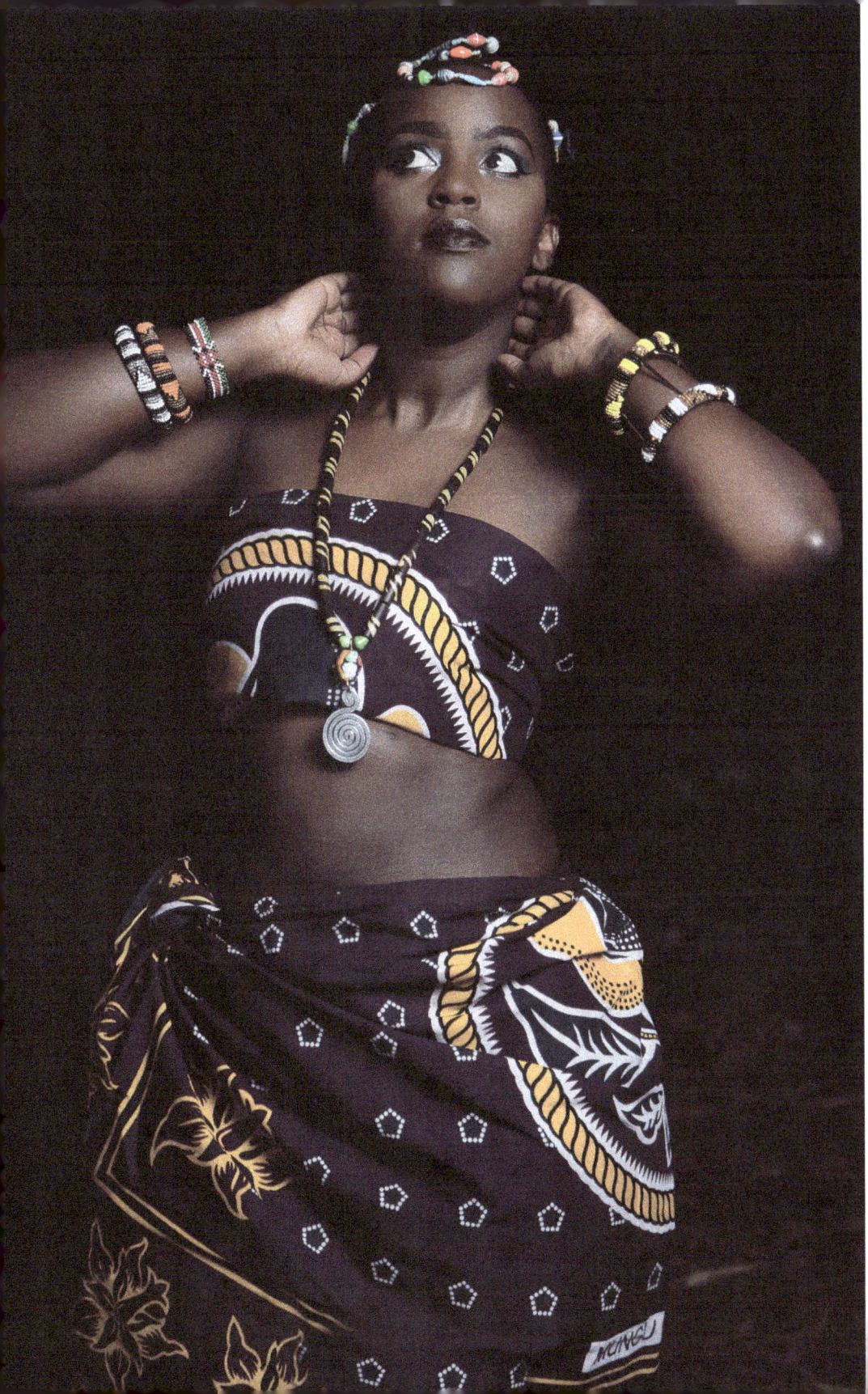

I call on You Sis...

...when the body changes are a
mystery to me, only you can reassure
me that this is normal.

Mother nature is a mystery. Older sisters are a source of wisdom. What advice would you give someone younger than you? Write down what that advice would be.

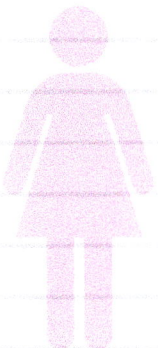

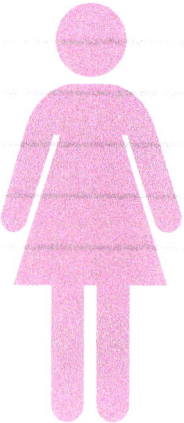

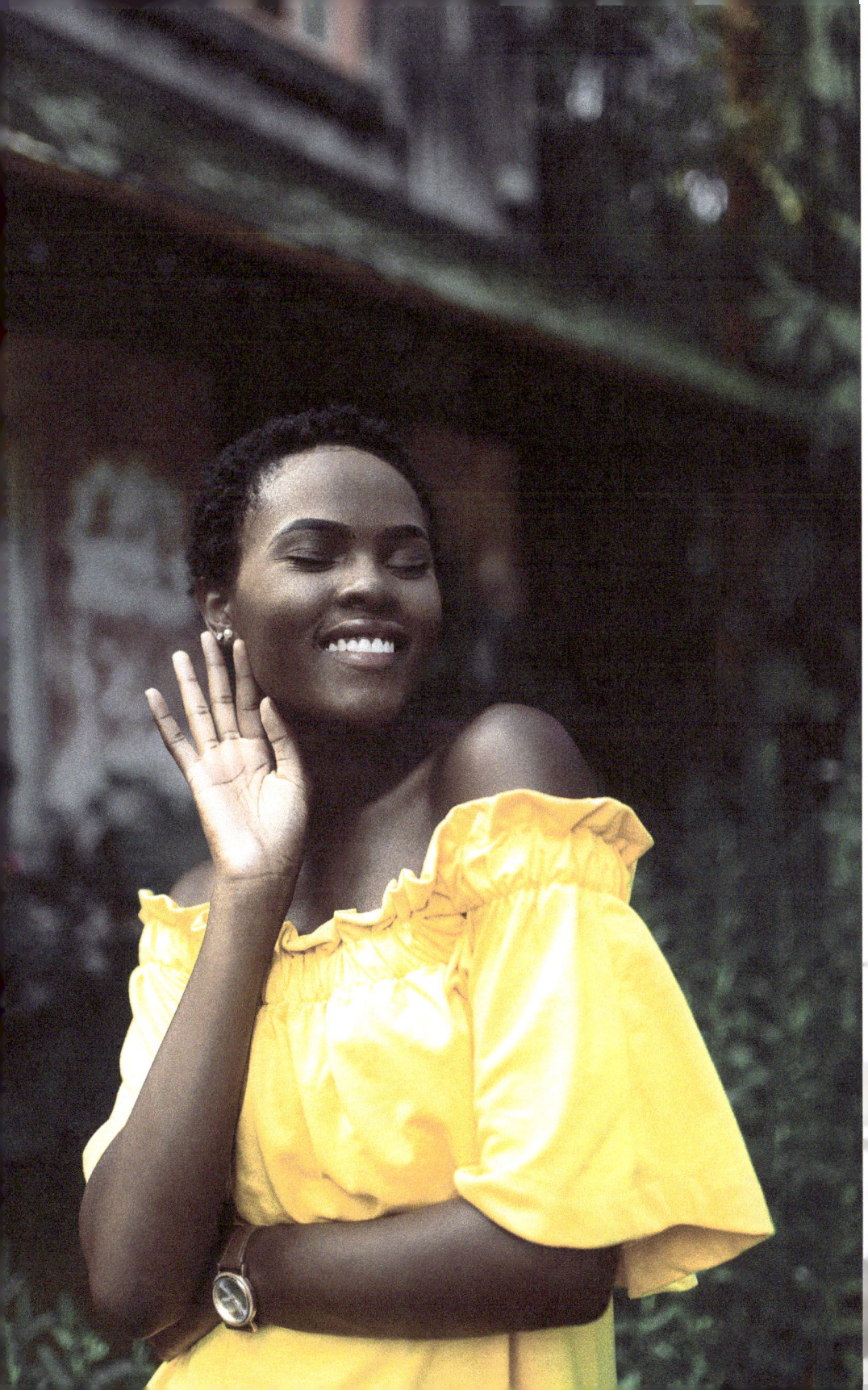

I call on You Sis...

...so I can be me, let my hair down, unwind, be myself, only YOU get me.

How grateful are you to have someone who gets you?
Write a letter to them thanking them for the role they
play in your life.

DATE:

"The greatest gift of life is friendship, and I have received ."
Hubert H. Humphery

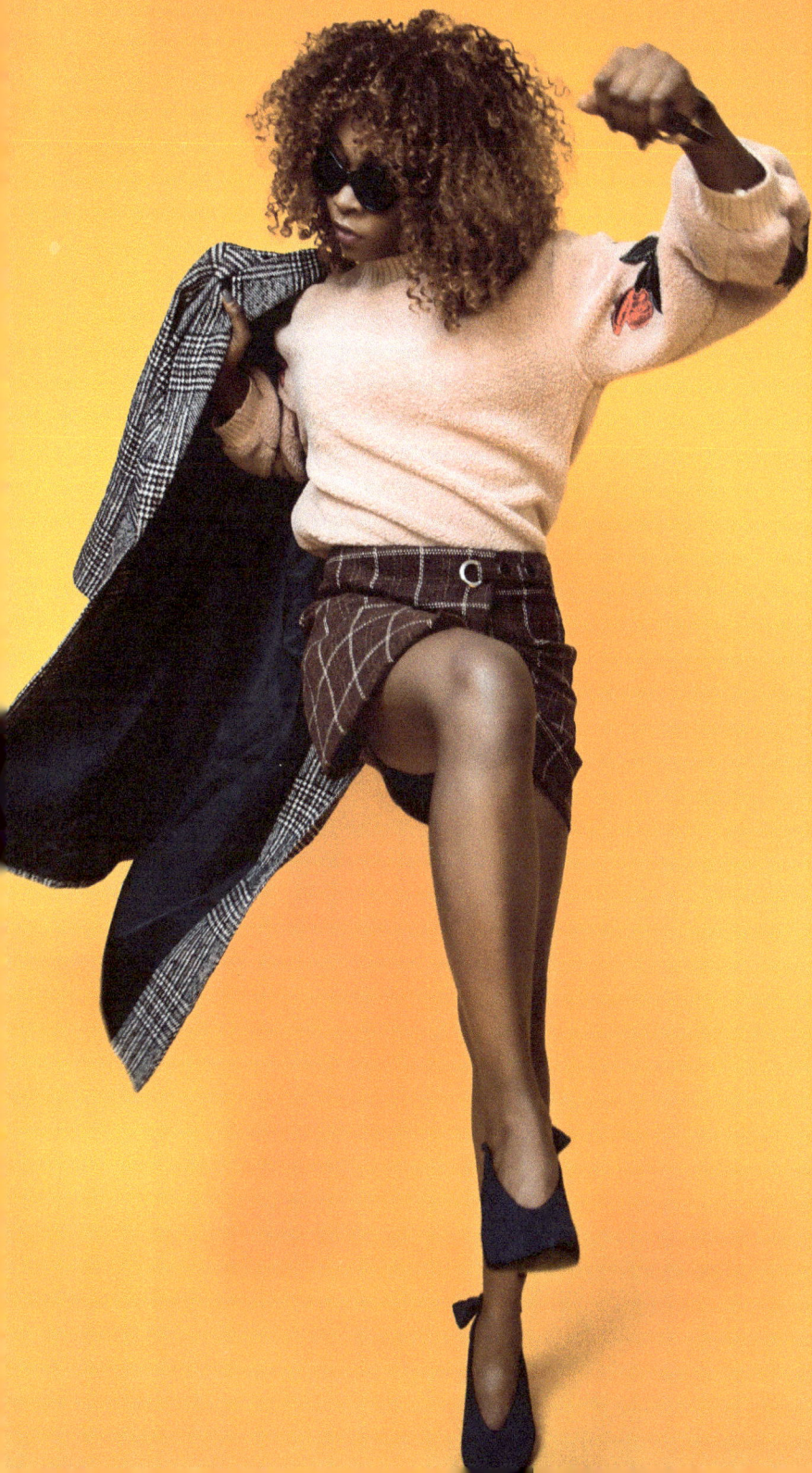

I call on You Sis...

...in my weakest moment, when my
spirit is low, for when I see you being,
I know I too can!

Who inspires you? whom would you like to emulate? Write about that person and why they inspire you.

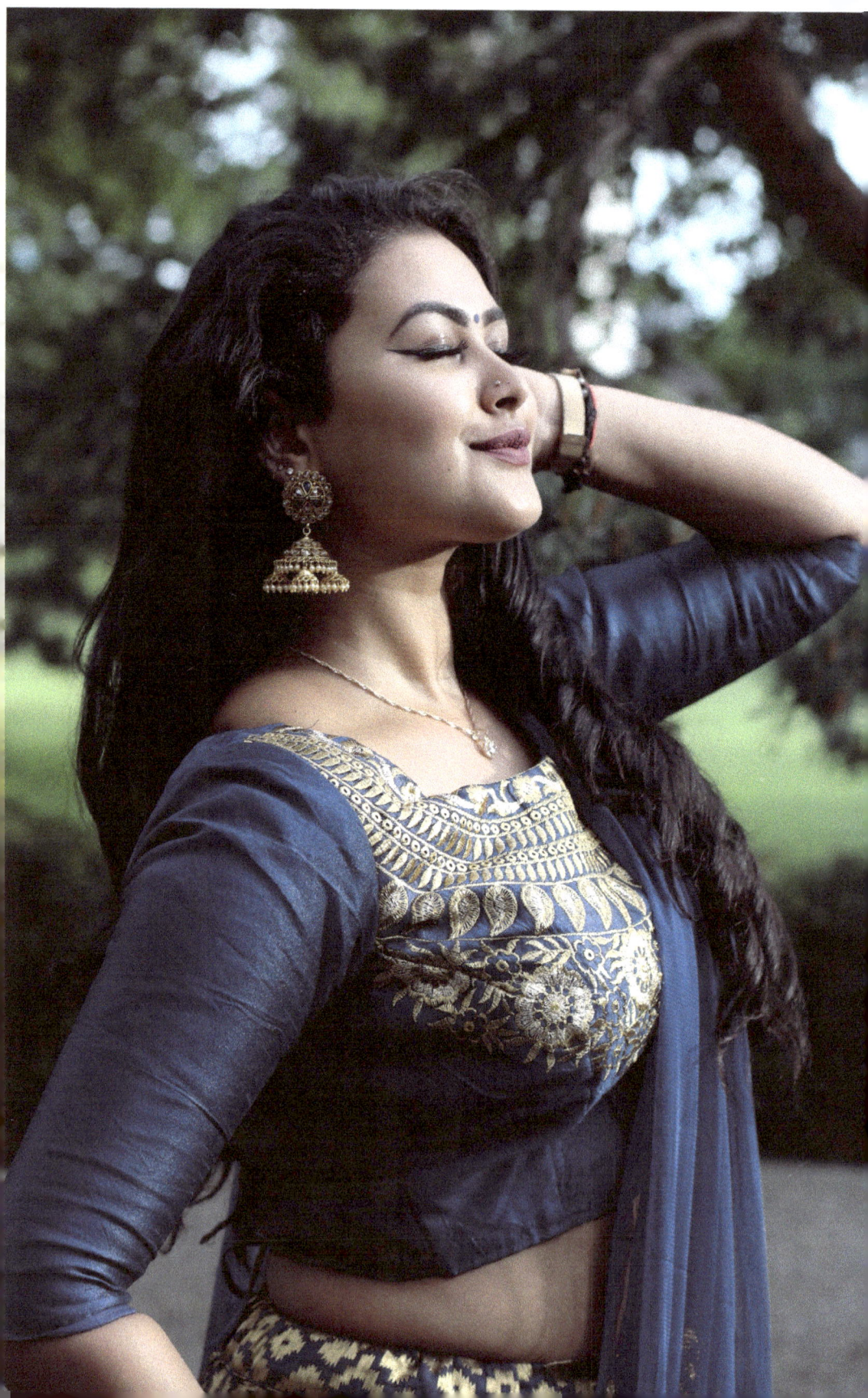

I call on You Sis...

...when alone I stand at a crossroads,
your voice directs me.

You are at a crossroads. Write about the choices you need to make. Write down options for these choices. Go deeper by writing the pros and cons of each choice.

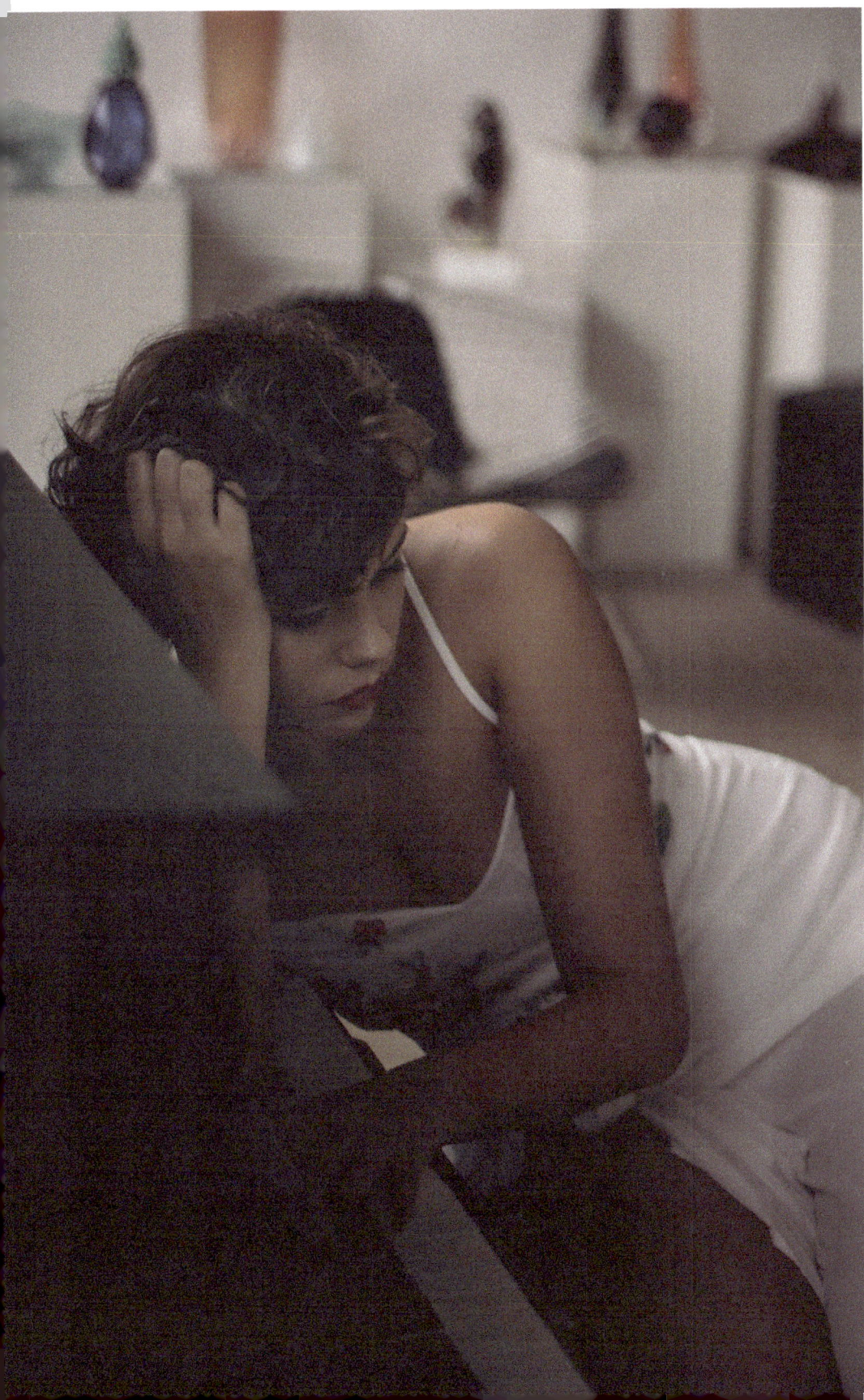

I call on You Sis...

...in my lonely moments, when I can't bear
the silence, you Sis, help me to understand,
I am never alone.

Loneliness can be depressing. Write about the roots of your loneliness and ways you can start to reach out to others. How can you form or join a community?

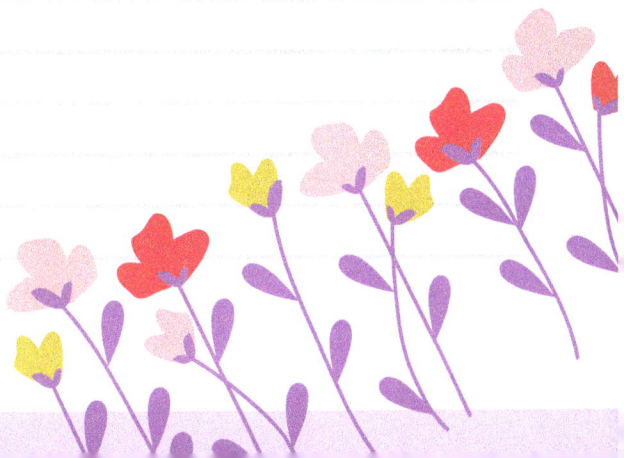

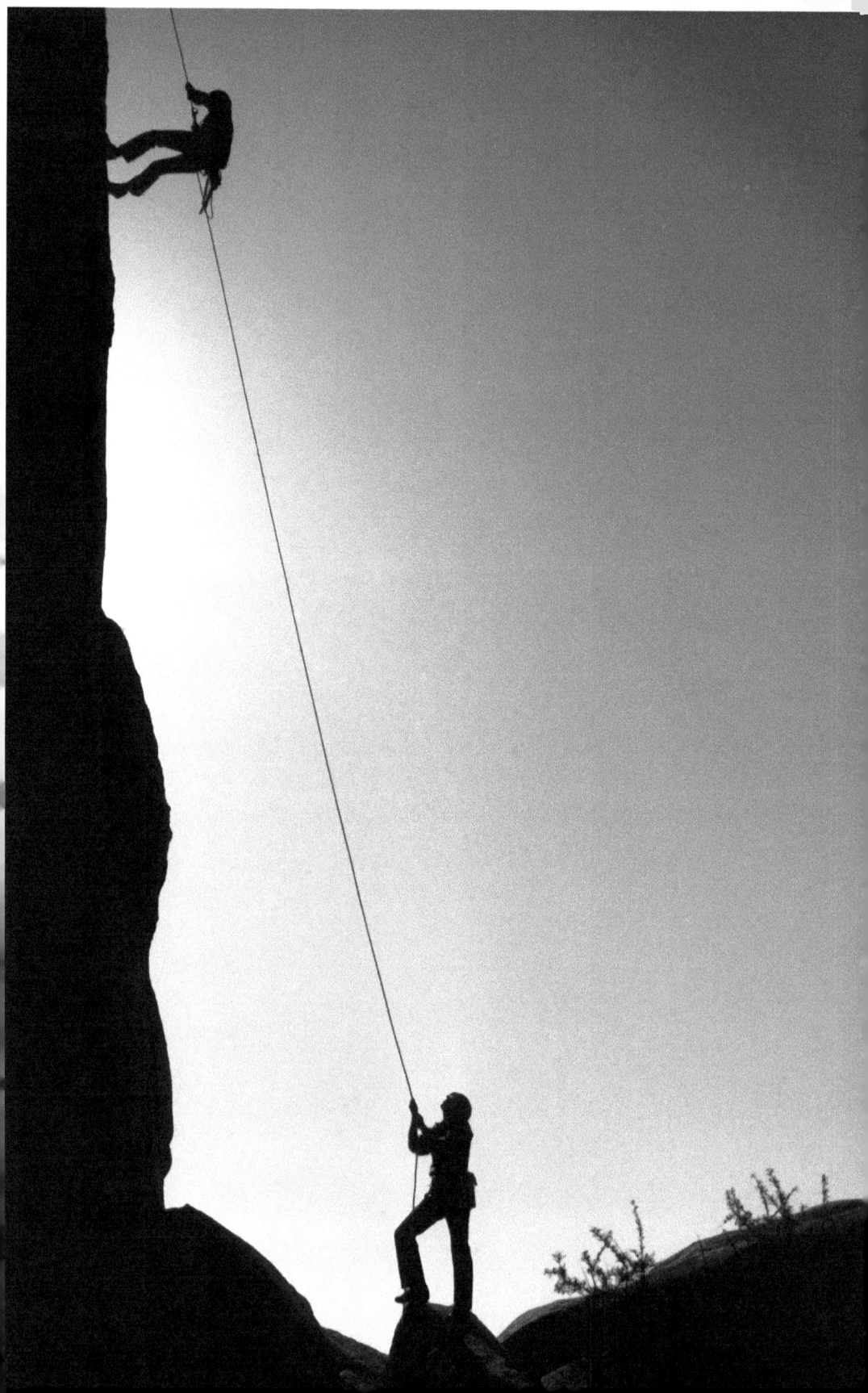

I call on You Sis...

...when my teenager seems to be
going astray, your voice maybe the
one he listens to.

There are no experts in Motherhood. It takes a village to raise a good citizen. What are some values and virtues you want to impart to your teenager? Write them down and share with a trusted friend who has frequent interaction with your child.

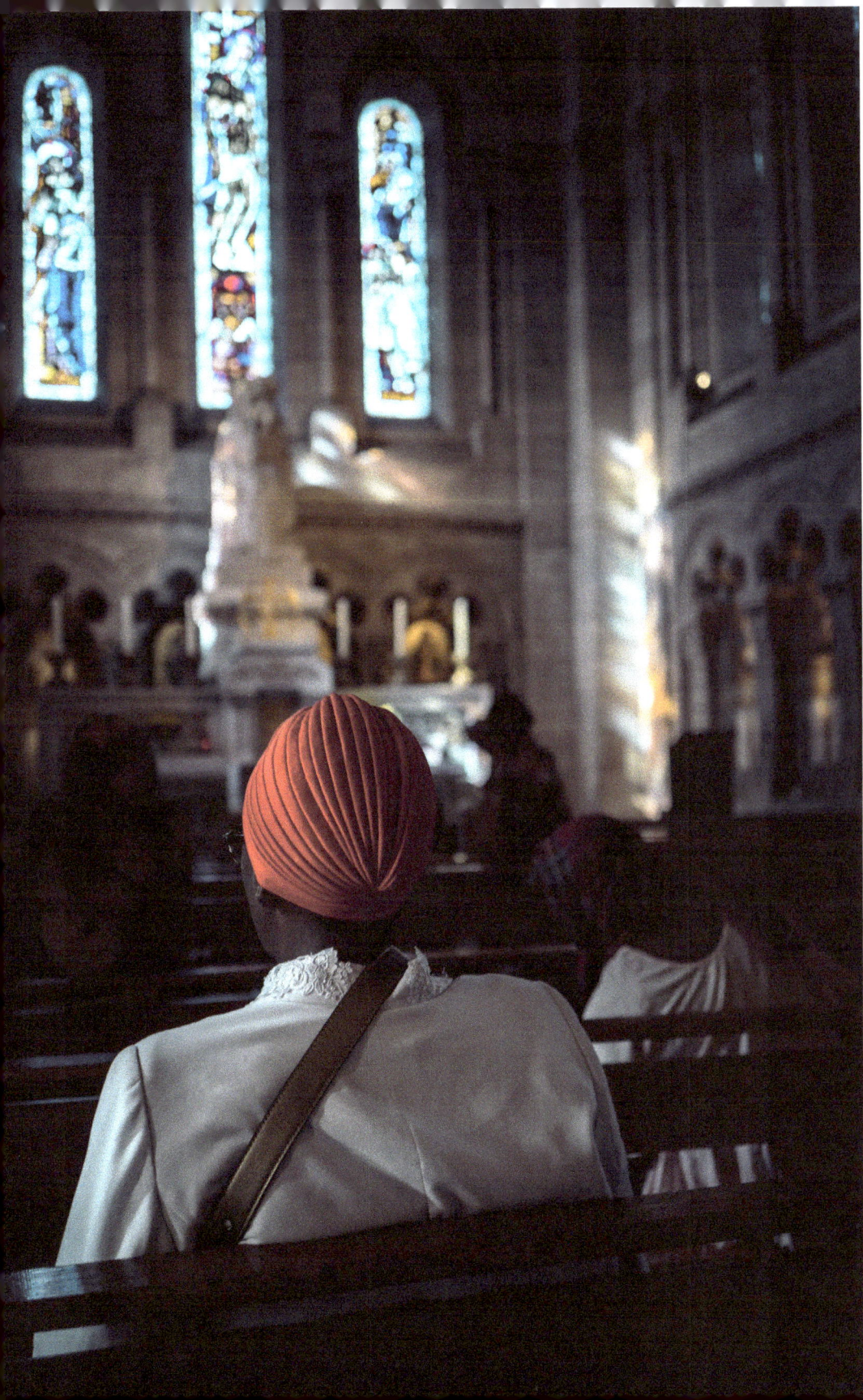

I call on You Sis...

...to kneel and pray with me, because
two are more powerful than one, and
there is no greater blessing.

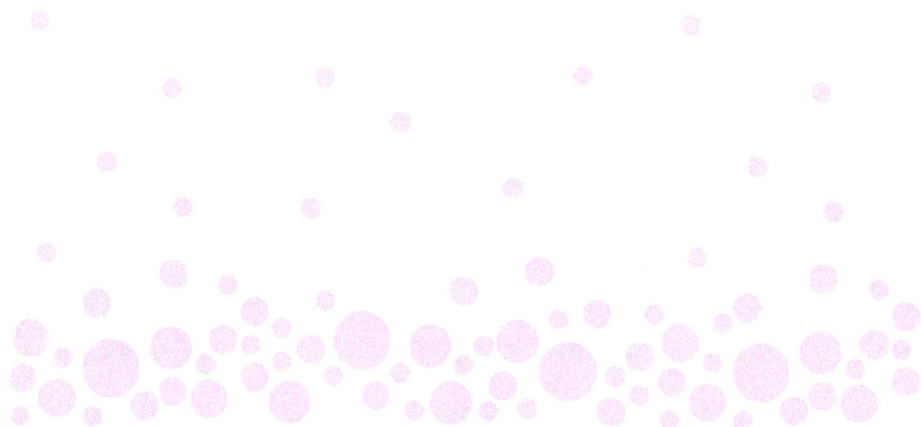

Faith is a great gift. It is the reason we get up every morning and face the day over and over again. Write about your faith and what it means to you.

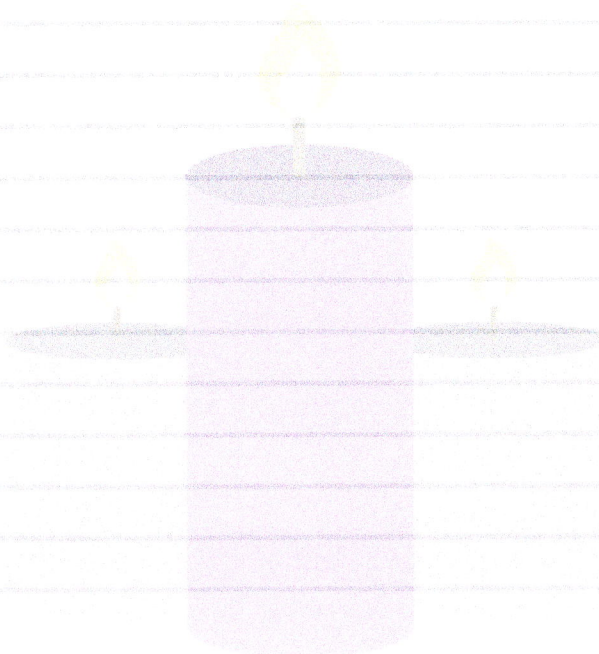

I call on You Sis...

...when my daughter/son decides to tie the knot. I call to share the joy, and of course you keep me from going overboard and making outrageous demands.

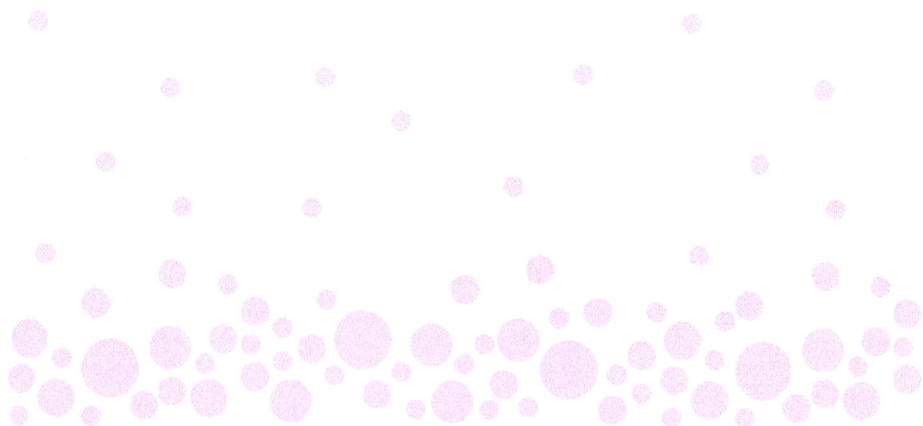

My joy is your joy, and these are our children.
Describe your joy for your children's future.

I call on You Sis...

...when at last I'm able to hold my baby in my arms, feel its heart against mine. Imperfect, but perfect to me. You my Sis, remind me that every child is perfect in God's eye, indeed a blessing.

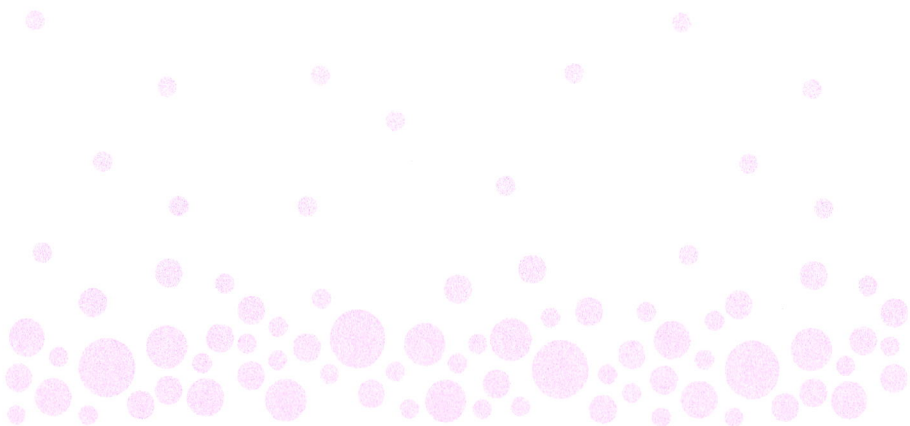

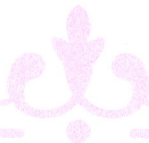

DATE:

Having a child with disabilities is one of the most difficult things a woman may have to face. How are you including these Sitsers and their family in your plans?

"I can't change the direction of the
wind, but I can adjust my sails to
always reach my destination."
Jimmy Dean

I call on You Sis...

...when I notice the faint positive strip on the pregnancy test, my heart sinks as the reason for my missed period is confirmed.

Not all pregnancies are celebratory moments. Offering reassurance and support no matter what the circumstances helps a Sister feel less lonely at this time. Plan your response here:

_____
_____
_____
_____
_____
_____
_____
_____
_____
_____
_____
_____
_____
_____
_____
_____

I call on You Sis...

...to stand beside me in the delivery room as I give birth. I bring new life, and I am immediately overwhelmed by the responsibility that lays on my shoulders.

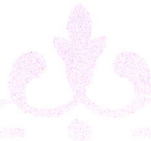

New life is magical, yet many experience the birthing process alone. Commit to be there for a Sister. If you're not invited, envision how a conversation with her might go, as you try to let her know that the birthing process is a divine miracle and social event.

Fertility issues can be isolating among friends. They can be difficult to understand. Listen without judging. Don't offer opinions. Ask how you can help. Visualize what you might say to a friend experiencing infertility.
Write down your visualization.

Your Sis knows the real you. You want her to anchor you. Write keywords she could say to keep you anchored. Share these with your Sis.

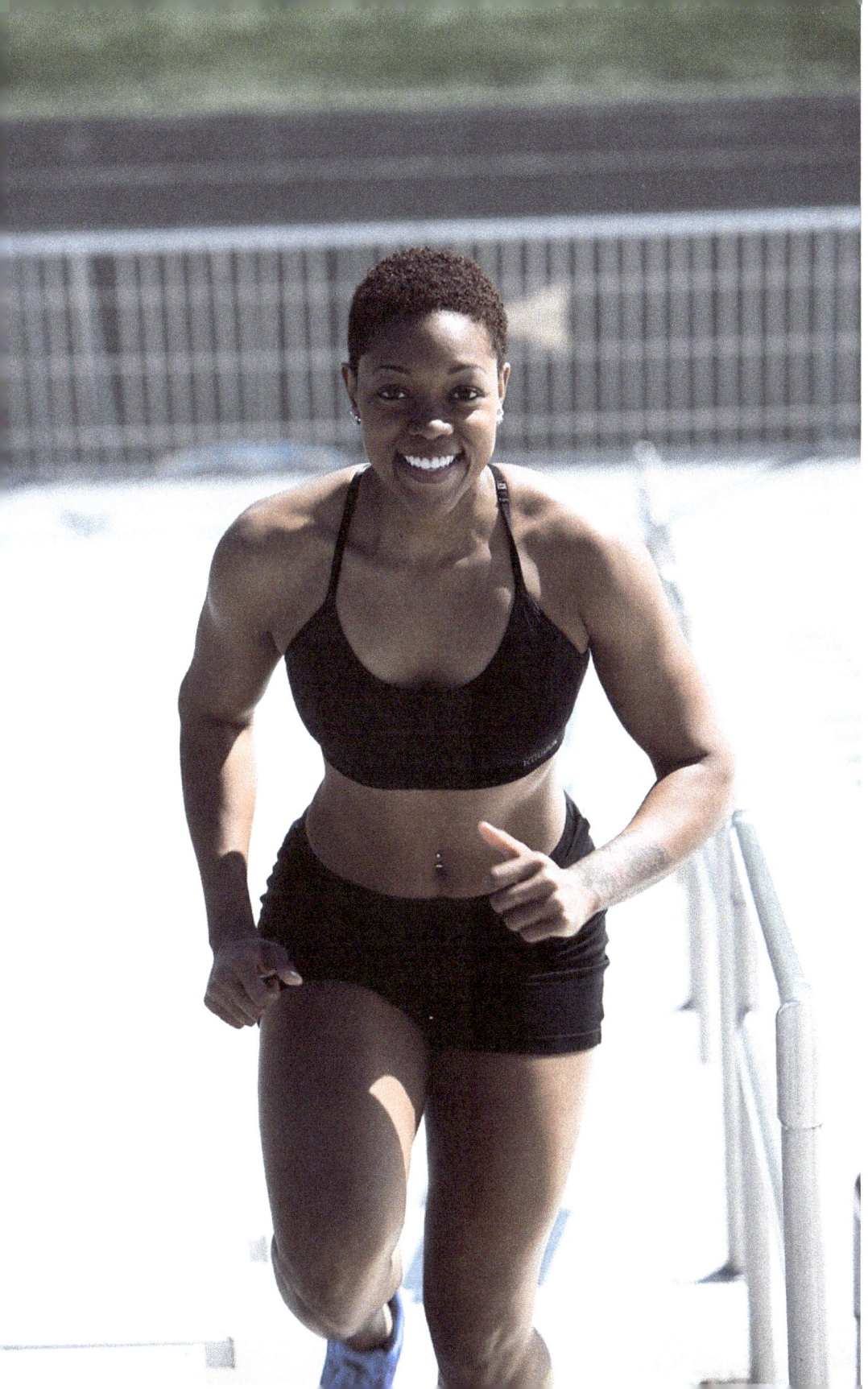

I call on You Sis...

...when I feel like giving up, you Sis help me
to stay positive and focused.

Giving up something you love or need can be soul crushing. Surround yourself with those that hold you accountable. Who are they? Write their names down. If you don't have any, write down the names of those you'd like to ask to be your accountability partners.

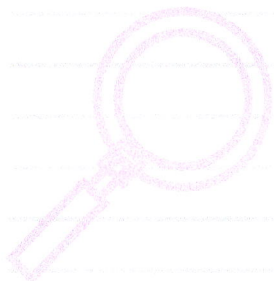

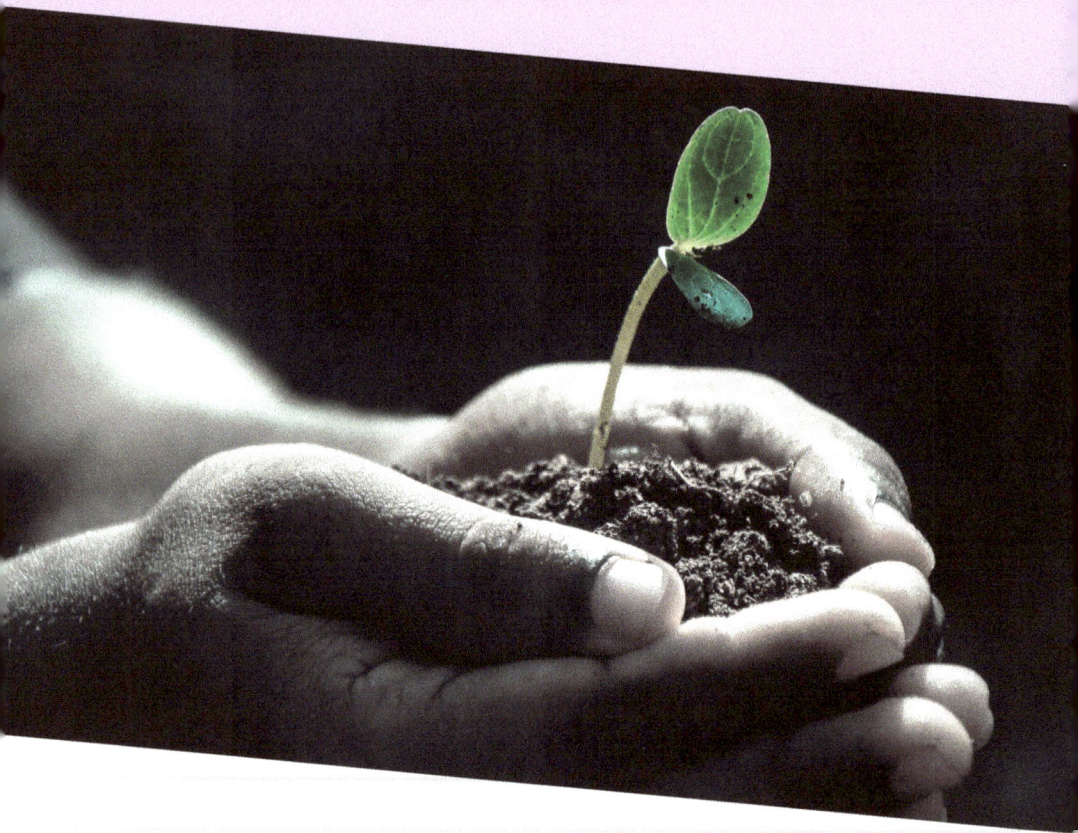

LIFE IS A JOURNEY, I CALL ON YOU TO
BE THE BEST YOU CAN BE FOR
YOURSELF AND OTHERS.

#ICALLONYOUSIS

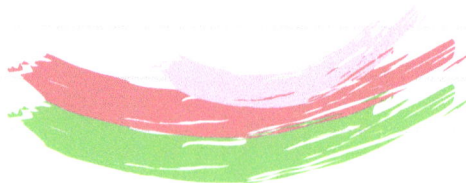

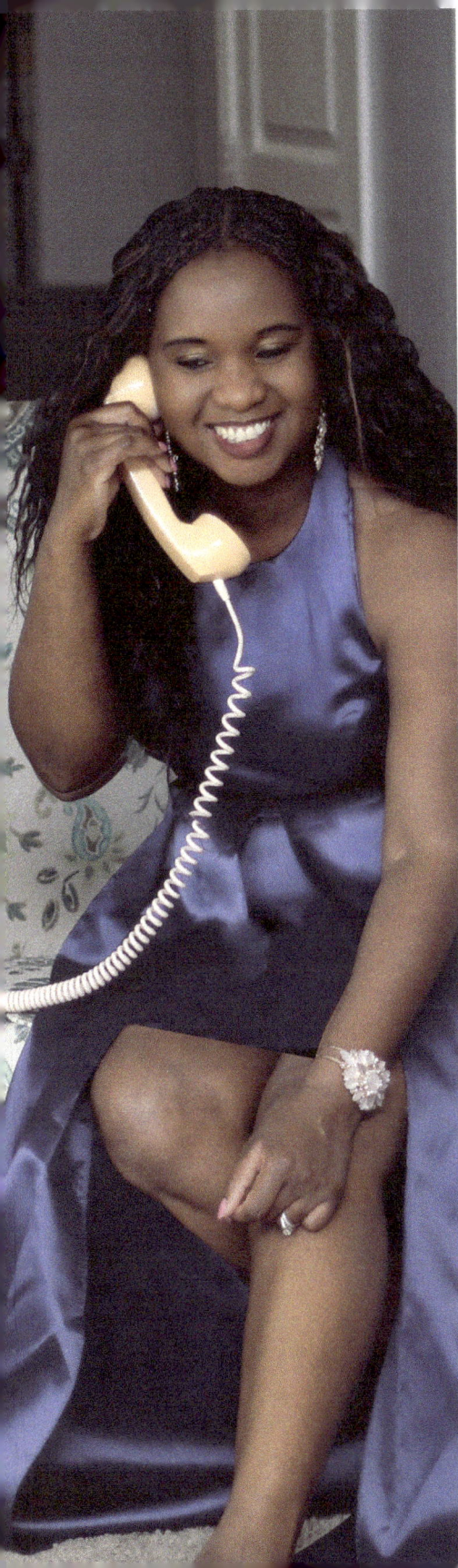

I wish you many pleasant sisterhood experiences in your life.

Because you answered the call from a sister to assist with the care and development of young sisters, please stay in touch. Reach out for speaking engagements and support Vasikana Project through these channels:

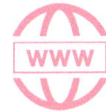

vasikanaproject.org

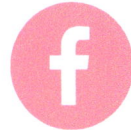

@vasikanaproject

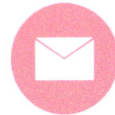

thevasikanaproject@gmail.com

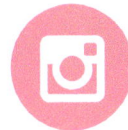

@vasikana_project